Buzz off
One man's fight
With Tinnitus

A
True story

By the author

Michael J Darracott

This book is published by
Michael John Darracott ©

A CIP record for this book
is available from the British library.

ISBN
978-1-4716-5146-5

Please visit my web site to see what other books I've published,
and for details of other books I'm still working on
that are near completion.

www.mikedarracott.com

PLEASE NOTE

The information, that you will come across within the pages of my book, are intended for informational purpose only.

Furthermore, under no circumstances is the information in these pages, to be used without your own Doctor, or any other Medical professionals, advice being obtained first. Were all different, and a lot of the information contained in this book could cause serious problems with your health. So please do not use anything mentioned in this book, until you have personally cleared it safe for yourself, with your Doctor, or other professional who cares for you. I cannot be held responsible, if you don't take notice of my written warning.

Chapter one

How it all started for me

One day while out shopping, I turned around, and was greeted with someone sneezing on me. Although I did not know it then, later this one chance incident would change my whole life forever. Within twenty four hours, I had the worse viral infection in my ears that I had ever had in my life. I awoke the very next day dizzy, and immediately knew something was very wrong, on trying to lift my head off the pillow the room began to spin around violently.

Furthermore, I was pinned to my bed with what felt like a downward force, this of course was because of the ear infection. I proceeded to try and get up, but was thrown back onto the bed; it was like I had come off a merry-go-round. I worked out that if I kept myself low to the floor, I could crawl to the bathroom without being sick or dizzy, but as soon as my head went a few inches upwards it all started up again.

After struggling to the bathroom, I had a heck of a job trying to pee, I had to kneel and relieve myself, and then crawl back to my bed, and just getting back into bed was hard, because I could not stand. I decided to stay in bed and wait it out, hoping it would subside, and it did after a few days, but I had the worse earache ever, and dreadful non - stop ringing sounds in both ears. I stayed in bed for the next four days, and when I felt I could actually stand up without the room spinning, my wife booked an appointment with our family doctor.

A few days later, I was sat in a surgeries waiting room, feeling so very dizzy, with very loud ringing sounds in both ears. Our doctor called my name, and I got up out of my seat and found it hard to walk straight. Let me explain, since I've had this disorder, when walking, I tend to lose balance. After a long examination of both my ears, the doctor said that I had suffered a severe ear infection, and that it's probable that the damage done would never reverse. He told me he would be booking an appointment for me with an ENT consultant (ENT is short for ears nose and throat).

When I got back home, the effects of the sounds in my head were driving me mental, non - stop noise that only I could hear, it was twenty four hours a day, every day. The dizzy attacks were constant, and when out walking I looked more like a crab, stumbling sideways. My hearing was well impaired, apart from the ringing sounds, I also could not hear that well now, like I use to. I looked forward to my up and coming appointment with the ENT specialist, and watched for the postman every day to deliver my appointment date.

Finally that particular letter came, and I was off to the hospital, on arrival I was weighed, and had my height recorded, and was told that I would be seeing the consultant later. In the meanwhile the nurse took me to a soundproof room to carry out a hearing test. In the room, I was told to place a pair of earphones over my ears, and was given a button to press every time I heard a different sound. I sat for about half an hour, and heard all manner of tones played, but guessed by the long breaks in between tones, that there were many I was not able to hear. I can recall a feeling of dread coming over me, because of the long waits between sounds; I knew this would mean gaps in certain sound frequencies, which I should be able to hear.

After the hearing test, the nurse printed off a couple of charts that had come out of the test equipment she had tested me with. Each chart was a recording of my ears performance. These she told me would now be passed to the consultant, and that he would see me shortly. After a short wait I was asked to go into room one, and was greeted with a kind warm welcoming smile from my ENT consultant. He asked me what had been going on; I told him that it all started with a severe viral infection in both my ears. He said that after reviewing my hearing test, it showed that I had a 40% hearing loss in my left ear and a 50% hearing loss in my right.

He then told me that the dizziness and balance problems coupled with the nonstop ringing sounds in both my ears, was because I have Meniere's disease, or endolymphatic hydrops. Furthermore, he said that the virus that I had caught, went straight to both my ears, and that I would be like this for the rest of my life.

He said that he was going to prescribe me a medicine called Serc 16©, and that it was a new drug, that was showing good signs of helping with balance problems associated with Meniere's disease. And that very little could be done with regards to the ringing sounds in my ears.

There is however some advanced treatments for the disorder, but I would not go for these unless I personally, was at the end of my limit. These are as follows, and please note always discuss your own medical problems with your own doctor. What I've written below was for my own use, and was what I learnt on my journey with the disease. Below I have listed some treatments, but check them up, because it's for info only, and I may well have got it wrong, but this is what I think the following procedures entail.

Endolymphatic sac shunt: Which entails an incision behind the offending ear, gives a fair chance of controlling dizziness, but you could suffer more hearing loss, spinal fluid leaking, further infection, and more unsteadiness to name a few complications Treatment as an outpatient.

Vestibular Nerve Section: This one entails an incision behind ear, and a stay in hospital, carry's a chance of improved hearing and control of dizziness, but also destroys the balance part of your inner ear, and can cause stroke and even death.

Intratypmpanic Gentamycin: which requires you to undergo around three treatments as an outpatient, treatment will be in eardrum, with a good percentage of help with dizzy spells, and hearing, but carries a risk of hole in tympanic membrane, and unsteadiness, and hearing loss. And it also destroys the balance part of your inner ear.

Labryinthectomy: procedure performed behind ear, a very good chance of regained hearing and a very good chance of help with dizziness, requires a stay in hospital, will destroy the balance part of your inner ear.

I have not gone for any of the above, instead I have been on Serc 16© for the last seven years, and have discovered many other ways of controlling my disease, of which I will share with you throughout the pages in this book. On return from appointment, I researched the options above on the internet, and decided the options were not for me, you could use the library if you don't have computer access. One day though, I may well get to the end of what I can take with this disease, and have no options left other than above ones already stated. Until then I will tell you all of what I have discovered about this disease I have, and share with you things I found that actually helped me.

The days of suffering non – stop dizziness and ringing sounds soon turned into months, so I was spending a lot of time consulting my doctor, who in turn told me at this time apart from the Serc 16 ©, there was not much else that could be done. I was told to go on the internet and join some support groups, and maybe do some **vestibular** rehabilitation **exercises**, and other things of which I will tell you about later in this book.

One clever little trick that can be performed, that's for the relief of ringing sounds in the ears, was the following, I found that it can work some time's,

Place both your hands over your ears, now move both your index fingers around to the back of your neck. You're aiming to be able to touch the area just below the skull in the nape of your neck. Next, with your ears closed over with your hands, start to use those fingers like drum sticks, you will hear the sound your fingers are making, if your ears are covered up. Continue to do this for around 2 to 3 minutes, and sometimes it can stop the ringing sounds. It does for me, it might not for you, but were all not the same, in any case check with your doctor if this is ok for you to try.

Well, my daily routine starts with awakening to the sound of ringing in both ears, every day now. I have tried doing the **vestibular** rehabilitation **exercises** throughout this period, and have not had much luck. I found that the feeling of sickness for me anyway, was just too much, so after around three months gave up on them. Below are some of the vestibular exercises that I did try that may be of use to you, but once again speak with your own doctor before trying anything in my book. I did get some benefit from the exercises overall.

Like I have written already, we are all individuals and these may help you, but you should ask your specialist or GP if they are ok for you to carry out. If your doctor says to try them out, it can be a great help for some with dizziness and balance problems. But check with your Doctor first.

Vestibular compensation:

This can allow the brain to regain some balance back, which in turn can reduce the effects of dizziness. You may have damage or an imbalance in both inner ear balance organs. Your body will have a constant fight, between the signals your brain are getting, and the position of your limbs, which will give rise to dizziness , sickness, and unbalance. I will now tell you of two of the exercises that I carried out for a while, starting with.....

Gaze stabilization exercises:

This exercise is intended to better your vision, and to make it easier for you to **look** at an **object that's stationary**, at the **same time moving your head**. Once again you should see your doctor or therapist, do not carry out any procedures in my book without seeking professional opinion first. If possible try to **gradually build** up the **speed** your **head moves** from **side to side**, but it's important that you **keep focused** on **the object**.

I also did the same exercise moving my head up and down while focusing on a stationary object, but if you become too dizzy maybe take a break or slow down a little. Keep doing it for maybe a minute or so, it can help to lessen your dizzy attacks.

Cawthorne-Cooksey exercises:

What these exercise's set out to do are the following, improve your general co-ordination skills, and help you in obtaining better balance generally. Will help bring about relaxation to the neck, and shoulder muscles, among other things. I find that any of above can help you regain balance, and reduce dizziness. You should first be assessed by a professional such as a therapist, to insure you learn to do the exercises correctly. And always consult your own doctor before embarking on any new health regime.

Typical exercises include:

Moving your eye's from side to side and up and down.

Looking at your finger at different distance's from your face.

Moving your head from side to side and up and down, while closing and opening your eyes.

While turning from side to side close and open your eyes or while bending forward or backwards.

I also tried walking with eyes closed, and then open, walking upstairs with eyes closed and back down again, but please proceed with caution of course. And have someone watch over you in case of a fall. Above are only a few of the exercises I carried out, you will find many more, ask your doctor or health care provider about these, and see if they are suitable for you.

If possible go for a nice walk every day, it's good for you, don't drink alcohol, it's bad for tinnitus and just makes it much worse, I will write a little more on that later. I know it's hard, but any type of exercise can really make a difference, as long as your doctor backs it. Always seek the advice of your own doctor, I cannot reiterate this enough, what's good for me, or anyone else, does not have any bearing on your own circumstances.

Later on in the book, I will list good foods, and bad foods for this disorder; I will also tell you of some foods I combine that actually stop my tinnitus for weeks at a time. Also coming up I will share with you the many things that I found on my journey both from friends, and on the internet. I hope I will be able to help you a little bit, with your suffering, and maybe, make you feel just a little bit more comfortable.

It's a horrid thing, waking up every day, to the sound of weird noises in your ears, that's if you got to sleep! No one around you can hear this, only you, so you feel isolated, and tearful. It drives you mad, day in day out, you can't escape it, these feelings are completely normal, were only human, but it's a tough life with this disease.

But if we share our experiences it makes it all a little bit more bearable.

That's what made me write this book, I felt the need to share my feelings with regards to my disease, with you the reader, write down everything I've had to endure so far. This disease came out of nowhere, and for quite a long time it took over my life, I now feel like I can control some aspects of it, and I hope that you may also come to control some aspects of yours.

From time to time, and for days on end, nothing works for me, none of my remedies, or even my Serc 16©, these for me are very dark days. Ones I find so hard to live with, they start off as a feeling of pressure in both my ears, and then ringing sounds start getting louder. Next, headache, a real bad one, that makes my stomach churn, all of this happens with the feeling of my ears and eyes trying to pop out my head. All of this can be coupled up with room spinning, dizziness, loss of concentration, and severe balance problems.

I of course turn to all my prop ups, but they don't work on these occasions, so it's an awful time, and I may well have to endure for several days. I don't know why the things I take work one day and not the next, but they do. And I'm glad that they do work some of the time, or I would really have a major problem. This is what this disease is like, it's quite a weird one to get your head around, I can get days of complete release from the grip of Meniere's disease, and then it's back as if it never went away.

I wish so much that I could go back to my life, the way it was before this black cloud called Meniere's disease, came along and stole it from me. I might sound melodramatic, but it's just so hard, the noise alone in your ears, drives you nuts, that's without all the other symptoms. You never know when it's going to decide to turn severe, so it's hard when planning any trips, or day to the day things.

I get very little relief, but when I get a day that's completely without ringing sounds in ears, or any other symptoms its bliss, but its overshadowed by the knowledge, that you know it will be back. I of course don't dwell on that fact, but nevertheless, it's very hard.

I have written the way my life is day to the day, what helped me to cope, and what I think should be avoided, in the hope that it may help you the reader, if you suffer from the same condition. I would urge you to seek permission, before you use, or carry out any of the things that I've written in this book, from your Doctor, or health professional, for your own safety first.

At the time of writing this book, I have now suffered eight years non – stop, with this disease, and it's the hardest thing in my life, apart from the death of my dad, who died in my arms from cancer, when I was only fifteen years old.

Chapter Two

Good food bad food

I will now concentrate for a moment, on the foods I found to be good for me with my condition, and which ones I avoid. I avoid salt at all cost; it always increases my ringing sounds and levels of unsteadiness. What does taking salt do to your tinnitus problems?, well, because Meniere's disease is actually, the result of an increase in fluid pressure inside of the ear, by reducing your own salt intake will reduce that fluid retention and subsequent pressure build-up. And also will help to maintain a better lower blood pressure, because too much salt can be bad for us with regards to healthy blood pressure. So seeing I've now had Meniere's disease for nearly eight years, I really reduced my salt intake.

Problem with our modern way of life, we don't cook so much fresh food, like we did many years ago, so a lot of the products we buy from the supermarket have high levels of sodium in. Thankfully for us though, the majority of supermarkets these days have labels that tell us the ingredients on most products we buy. So I always look for the lowest sodium content items, and make a habit of buying fresh foods when possible, which tend to be low in salt or have no salt at all.

Five a day is the way; I always eat lots of fresh fruit and vegetables every day, and drink lots of water. I drink quite a bit of water, it increases urinating, and this in turn can help to lower salt levels in your body, which I find can reduce my ringing sounds in my ears. But, please consult your own doctor before embarking on anything that I do, it's about you, not me, so be sure to follow up with your doctor. Sometime like all of us, I eat a little bit too much salt by mistake, and the ringing sounds in my ears increase to deafening levels, that's when I drink a couple of cups of water, and when I have a wee, it helps to get the excess salt out of my system. Or you could go for a nice walk, exercise will make you sweat, and this will help to lower the salt in your body through sweating.

When I first started walking every day, it killed me, I have other problems that are disabling you see, so I force myself to walk quite a long distance each day, to reap the benefits it brought. In my case, I found that walking slowly each day built up a little bit of extra muscle on my legs, this in turn helped to buffer some of the pain. Furthermore, like already written about, the fact that walking was making me sweat, I also found that this was removing excess salt from my body. I must stress talk to your own doctor, what I do works for me, and I do this because some of the foods I eat still contain low amounts of salt, and I try to regulate the amount left in my body.

So anyway, by simply walking I knew I could lose some of the excess salt in my body through sweating; this in turn reduced the amount of fluid building up in my ears, which in turn reduced some of the ringing sounds caused by the fluid in my ears. On return home I would take a couple of glasses of water, to rehydrate my body, and this of course led to having to wee, which further helped to remove any excess salt from my body, and more importantly from my inner ears. My fitness regime works well especially when I've overindulged in too much salt. But this like I say works for me but may not work for you, your body is unique to you, so consult with your own doctor.

I found out on the internet, that increased blood flow, especially in the ears, can help to decrease tinnitus, and dizziness. So I put some of the suggestions I found on the internet to the test, with me being the guinea pig so to speak. Below are some of the easy to find, and buy to items, that I use daily in my fight against dizziness and ringing sounds in both my ears.

Lemons:

I heard that if you grate the zest off a lemon and eat it, that it can stop the ringing sounds in your ears. Furthermore, it was because of the bioflavonoid that's in the zest of the lemon that helps to reduce the tinnitus. So the very next day I was off to the greengrocers to by me some lemons ☺☺ when I got back, I got my grater out, and proceeded to very gently grate just the tangy zest of a single lemon onto a plate.

I scooped this up into a spoon, and swallowed it using a glass of water, it was not the best taste in the world, but it was not that hard to get down. I was totally surprised that within 4 hours of taking this, my ringing sounds in both my ears just stopped completely for the first time in years. I was so very excited and happy; I could not believe that this had occurred; I had found a way to stop the dam ringing.

The next day I awoke and my ears were still silent, I rushed down the stairs, got a lemon out of the fridge and repeated the process. For the next 5 days I had no ringing sounds, it was amazing, but on the 6th day the ringing sounds just came back for no reason, and the lemons would not work anymore. I stopped taking the lemon zest, I was so upset that it worked for a short while, and then stopped working. But as my ringing sounds in my ears continued to give me a life of absolute hell, I decide to try the lemons again, and just like before they stopped the ringing in just a few hours.

I have no idea why it works for a while, and then stops working, but it does work for me, so this is one of my weapons against the ringing sounds in my ears, you may have buzzing sounds, or other types of sound, people with tinnitus will have all types of weird sounds going on. Check with your doctor before trying anything I have written in this book, I can't over emphasize this point enough, so sorry if I repeat myself. I think what happens is that the bioflavonoid that's in the lemon, increases blood flow to the ears, which in turn reduces the fluid building up within the inner ear, thus reducing the tinnitus. Like I said it works for me, so I am very happy about this, and will continue to include the zest of lemons in my daily diet. I am trying to find a source for lemon bioflavonoid, without having to use Lemons.

Zinc:

I take zinc, I buy it from most chemists or health shops, and I found that it can reduce the ringing sounds I suffer with, because of my Meniere's disease. I only take the amount it says on the packet; it's not as good as the lemons but works for me. I take this these days with the lemon zest, and most of the other stuff I will be writing about here all at once. But like already stated, please check with your own doctor before embarking on anything you hear about, both here in my book, or anywhere else. Zinc can be found in foods such as, eggs, beans, lamb, pumpkin seeds and oysters.

Ginkgo:

This supplement widely available from health stores or the chemist is said to work because it increases the blood circulation anywhere in your body, and in my case, it's the increase of blood, which my inner ears get, that I believe gives a reduction of the ringing sounds in both of them.

MSM Methylsufonylmethane:

I started out on MSM (Methylsufonylmethane) because I heard it was good for joint pain. I took some, and it really works so well for my bad back, knee, and neck injury, but to my amazement, it also helps to ease tinnitus. I had a very good reduction in my ringing sounds in both of my ears while using MSM, but was advised by a friend to take it for say around 8 weeks at a time. Because, in some people it can cause some unwanted symptoms. I myself, have never had any problems taking this, and have read many good reports with regards to this, from other people taking it. It also can be obtained from all good health shops. Seeing that it may cause the odd weird symptom in some people, I now take one tablet a day, and after 8 weeks, then stop taking it for a week.

Apple Cider vinegar:

I also found out that if you buy apple cider vinegar, and dilute with some water, that it can also reduce the ringing sounds in your ears. So I brought a bottle of it, got 3 tablespoons of the vinegar, mixed it with a half pint of water and drank it. I was having a real bad attack of ringing in the ears at the time, and it stopped it within 2 hours. It was however quite hard to get down as you can imagine, so it's not surprising that some people can't stomach it, but it worked. But check with your doctor, my ringing sounds have persisted for 8 years, every day 24 hours a day, so anything that works, gives me my life back. I must stress however, that nothing that I take works for ever, but many of the preparations and supplements, foods, can work for weeks, months, days or just hours, for me.

Try to eat as many healthy foods as possible, to name just a few, poultry, eggs, pasta, yogurt, fresh fruit and vegetables daily, fish, bread whole grain, hard cheddar cheese, use olive oil, celery, lemons, potatoes, garlic. Try to cut back or eliminate the consumption of cow's milk, and dairy products, alcohol, sugar, and try to lower caffeine intake such as tea or coffee, cola. This list is not exhausted by any means, but it made a big difference to the management of my tinnitus. But check with your own health advisor or doctor, remember, were all different, and we all have to be sure what we take, is going to work with our own regime, better to be safe than sorry.

I would like to pass on some information that's not about my tinnitus, but feel it may be of help to anyone out there who suffers with high blood pressure. I went for a routine checkup with my own doctor, and after my examination, he declared that I had high blood pressure. I could have been knocked down with a feather at this news, because in the last 25 years of going regularly to the doctors, my blood pressure had been perfect. So I was told it was up by 15 points, in the bad zone so to speak, so I was very worried. He told me, that he wanted to put me on the conventional drugs for lowering blood pressure. I said that I was not sure about it, because in the back of my mind, I remembered a lot of friends having told me that they had not got on well with these types of drugs, so I asked for an alternative.

He weighed me and said I was about 12 pounds overweight for my build, and said that if I can lower my blood pressure by losing some weight that I would not have to go on the drugs, so I agreed to give it ago. When I got back home, I went on the internet and checked up about high blood pressure. I found out quite a few things that you can eat, that are said to naturally lower blood pressure, and here are just some of the ones, which are said to maybe lower high blood pressure.

Celery: As been mentioned to help lower blood pressure, its thought that the substance called Apigenin, that's found in celery is good for your heart and also helps to lower your blood pressure. So I started to eat a couple of sticks of the stuff a day.

Raisins: Lower blood pressure, Keep blood healthy and improve your digestion, also helps to lower your cholesterol levels.

Bananas: Contain high amounts of potassium, and are and excellent way of lowering your blood pressure.

Melons: Also contain high amounts of potassium, and are and excellent way of lowering your blood pressure. Other foods that I eat that are good for lowering blood pressure are...........

Tomatoes: Prunes: Oranges: All have quite high levels of potassium in them, and I eat them every day. The list once again is far from complete, but I certainly eat these each and every day.

And for me it worked☺☺, and like I wrote before, I started walking a lot, and coupled this with eating all of above for around 6 months. I went back to the doctor, and found that I had lost a stone in weight, and that my blood pressure was now totally normal. All above was achieved simply by sensible weight loss, and eating above items within my normal diet. It was a very happy day for me, and I hope that if your doctor advises you that above will be a good thing for you to try out, that it works for you too. Just be sure to consult your doctor about anything I have written before trying it.

I live every day hoping for a cure, but until that day comes, I will continue to do my level best to research and find any new ideas, or diets that might allow me to live a normal lifestyle. I know what it's like, many times a week I don't get any sleep, I just lie in my bed trying to block out the sounds that are in both of my ears. Furthermore, I then have to face a whole day with the same sounds and pain. It's so hard; you're alone with this, because of course you're the only that can hear it. In the early days of my disease, I thought like we all do, that it was just some kind of bad flue, or something, and that it would pass off. But, by the end of my first full week, I was going mad, and found myself so very depressed, that I was crying my heart out, not knowing what to do. If this sounds like you, don't be scared, there's a whole lot of people out there just like us, join a group, share your problem, it helps.

I went completely downhill in the beginning; I would find what I hoped to be a cure, just to find out later it did not work. And of course I would pick myself up, and look harder for something else that might alleviate the pain, and the sounds, and dizziness. But time and time again, it was just a hopeless quest, leaving me even more worn out, and a little bit more depressed. There is no cure at the time of writing this book, but there are things that can help you limit the impact it as over you. What I would say to anyone reading this with the same disease, would be, don't surrender, never give in, you can't beat anything in life this way, confront it square on. Furthermore, it's only a human response do feel alone, and wonder why it's happened to you, tearful even, once you get over these initial feelings, I found it easier to take my disease on. I tend to concentrate on anything that improves my condition even in the smallest way, and then nurture it, to its full potential, and then add some other thing that also improves it.

It's a great feeling to fine a process, or food, or anything, which actually lessens the symptoms of this extremely full on disabling disease, known as Meniere's disease. It's one of the worse things that as happened to me in my life, and after living with it now for nearly 8 full years, It's almost like I was born with it, because of the length of time its raged on. I would give anything to be rid of this, but I am as far as the medical fraternity are concerned, in the area of, (I will have to live with it ☹) or have an operation that could leave me worse off in my particular case.

Getting back to the foods that I take from above list, although they don't cure the disease, in my case it gives me periods of no ringing sounds, of which I can attribute to the taking of the foods above. Furthermore, in my case, I found that walking each and every day, as also lowered my blood pressure, and as made me feel much fitter generally, I also have a much healthier appetite. A lot of the food I eat is very good for the heart, and circulation, so that's a bonus. I try very hard to only concentrate on the positive sides of my daily regime. And try to block out any pain, or negative feelings that the disease ultimately puts me through, some days I win, others I lose.

In the next chapter, I will list a lot of the devices, and aids, I've tried, and tell you how I got on with them. Please remember that I am writing about myself, and that I am in no way stating this is good for anyone. Once again, I would like to reiterate, that were all different, and that it's safer to ask your doctor, or health care provider, if anything that I've written in this book that helped me, is safe for you to try.

I would also like to state, that the hearing aids I have to wear, have helped a little to block out the ringing sounds in my ears. But only by masking them with the sound of the crackle the miniature speakers make, and enhancing external sounds. Ironically, these sounds are also irritating, but are somewhat different sounds, to the ones I'm forced to endure with my disease, so in a weird way give me a break. I don't know if you the reader, wear hearing aids, but you may well feel the same way as I do, I only wear my hearing aids when in a very noisy public place. Because, I find with the nerve damage in my ears, and the ringing sounds, coupled with certain tones, and frequencies, that I can no longer hear, so for me the hearing aids help a little bit.

Chapter Three

Getting Techi

Pillow speakers:

Well like everything else in life, the technical revolution as arrived in nearly all areas, so tinnitus products are in abundance. One of the first gadgets I tried out on myself was a tinnitus pillow speaker, which is simply a pillow with speakers built into it. There are many types on the market, and of course with different prices to choose from; the one I used was fitted with an mp3 connection, so you can listen to your favorite sounds. And I recall it cost around £30, which was money well spent. The speakers are well hidden, and don't give any bulges in the pillow where your head rests, my wife was not disturbed by the sound it made either.

You will probably know by now, that when you're in a quiet environment, especially in bed at night, that your tinnitus sounds are very loud, and that this will make sleeping so very hard. If you're like me, you would have spent most of the day listening to the constant noise of tinnitus, and will be so tired by now, but now you face a restless night. It works by distracting you from the sound of your tinnitus, and eventually the sound of your tinnitus subsides into the background, and you finally fall to sleep. I found it to be a worthwhile ally in aiding me to a restful peaceful sleep.

The aim with listening to another sound is to insure that the new sound is not louder than the actual tinnitus; the new sound you hear must be lower than that of the tinnitus one you hear. By using this method, you can eventually train your brain, to become a little bit less aware of your tinnitus, which is what using other sounds aims to do. Test out different sounds until you find one you're happy and comfortable with. Using any sound type gadgets, you always need to insure, that you can still hear your tinnitus, simply masking out the tinnitus with another sound will not work, your brain still needs to be able to hear the sound of your tinnitus, to enable it to make it fade away eventually.

Sound generator:

You can buy a device called a sound generator, or a white noise generator; they can be worn like a hearing aid. The prime use of these is the same as above, which is to help you fade the unwanted annoying sounds of your tinnitus eventually hopefully away, by playing you a pleasant sound, that's more pleasing to you. After a short while your brain will home into the pleasant sound that you choose to hear over the tinnitus one, and eventually may even stop the tinnitus sound for a period. I used these, and after wearing them, and concentrating on the sounds I chose, I found that many times after turning off the sound generator, my tinnitus sounds at either stopped altogether, or at least, faded away to hardly hearing it. But you still need to have the volume set so it won't drown out your tinnitus sound completely, and eventually your tinnitus sounds will hopefully fade away.

Hearing aids:

I wrote earlier about the use of hearing aids, I find that when using mine, they increase the normal sounds I wish to hear, which in turn help to fade out the tinnitus sound I don't wish to hear. I think this is a very good way of getting an instant break, from that same old tinnitus sound that we are forced to listen to day in day out. Another thing I would like to touch on is being anxious or stressed by tinnitus, this will lead to an increase of the symptoms, and I have found this to be the case with my own disease. To combat that, I do a series of deep breathing, and keep my heart rate down, and try to relax as much as possible.

The main thing with this disease for me, is to watch my diet, eat good fresh foods, lower salt intake, and alcohol, caffeine, and sugar to name a few, this made a big difference for me. Coupled with the exercise that I've already wrote about, and walking each day, I can now win breaks from the sounds in my ears. But I can never stop my constant fight against my own disease, because it's there all the time, I have learned to manage it with what I've wrote in this book. Below I will continue with the gadgets that I have used and know of.

Ear plugs:

Ok, I know, not much of a gadget, but a loud noise, a siren, any type of loud noise can make your tinnitus sounds rise to such a high volume, that it's truly disabling. So carry a pair at all times, so if you hear a real loud noise, put your ear plugs in, they might just save you a severe episode.

Above are the gadgets I use daily, when I need to, there are more on the market, but I only use the ones above, so have no real experience of any other ones. But you will find one that works for you, it's just a matter of research, and trial and error, but like me I am sure you will find a gadget or two. This chapter is a small one, because I get a lot of results from diet and exercise, coupled with my supplements.

In the next chapter I will tell you my daily regime, from start to finish, but as always would stress what I do might not be good for you, so please consult with your own doctor or health worker. I am sorry to repeat this over and over, but it's a real important thing from your point of view.

I hope by writing out my story, to help people with the same disease, to stand up and let them know, that I'm another one of millions of people out there, suffering with the same horrible symptoms, and that were not alone. And I hope that many of you out there find something in my book that helps you just a little, or hopefully a lot.

My own story, has been an 8 year long one, and I still can't believe that I am sat here in the year 2012, writing about a disease that started so long ago for me. Furthermore, by writing this, I feel like I've finally really come to terms with the fact, for me that is, that I may never get better. But I do think that I have tamed it, and at times win complete weeks of freedom, away from the noise in my ears.

I think we all have it within us, to go out and seek out something to help ourselves, it may just be support, or a friendly ear, or a shoulder to cry on, but what I call it is hope, hope that one day we will win, and that were once again as we would like to be. If we lose hope, then we have already lost, keep going, keep hoping, searching, it's good for the soul. Keep your chin up; because there really are people worse off than us.

Chapter Four

My daily routine

The alarm goes off, it's another day, after a shower its breakfast, I have a bowl of unsalted muesli and a cup of decaffeinated tea. With my breakfast, I take one Serc 16 tablet ©, one Ginkgo biloba tablet, one Zinc tablet, 1 garlic oil tablet, one MSM tablet.

I also find drinking one small bottle of Yakult©, is very good for my digestion, so I wash all my tablets down with it. Next, I go for a walk with our dog Marley, and on return back home, set about writing my books.

Around Mid - Morning, I take a small handful of dried cranberries, and a small handful of dried Raisins, with a glass of water. Around Mid – Day, I have a glass of water, and a banana, and then walk our dog Marley again.

Late afternoon dinner around 5.15 pm, I have any number of things; some days chicken, some - day's fish, but always keep the salt content as low as possible. If possible, I aim to get my salt from naturally occurring sources, and not to buy any foods that are processed with added salt. We all need some salt to live of course, so I have not removed eating it altogether.

After dinner we take Marley for another walk and on return home around 7 pm, I have a cup of decaffeinated tea, and I eat a banana and an apple. For supper, around 10 pm, I have a further cup of decaffeinated tea, and maybe a plain biscuit.

During the week, especially when I'm having a real bad one, if my ears have increased ringing sounds, then I will start a course of Cider Apple Vinegar as already written earlier in this book. If that does not help to reduce the ringing sounds, I will take the lemon remedy I also wrote about earlier. Furthermore, during a prolonged attack, I also eat a stick of celery or two, and drink a little more water than usual, to make me wee a bit more. The weeing helps remove any access of salt that I may have accidently taken, which in turn gave me an increase in my tinnitus.

If none of my remedies above don't work, which for me is very rare, I will increase my walking to also burn off any excess salt in my body, especially with in the inner ear. I would like to remind you all again, that we are all different, and please see your own doctor, or health care provider before attempting anything new.

You may be wondering what supplements, and foods, work best at stopping my tinnitus, and dizziness, as well as good for keeping blood pressure down. I would say **for me** the following really work well, and I've given them all a mark out of ten, with ten being very good. These are the ones I think are the best for me.

Lemons:	8 ☺	
Celery:	4 ☺	
Bananas:	7 ☺	
Garlic:	8 ☺	

Raisins:	7 ☺
Ginkgo:	10 ☺
Serc 16 ©:	10 ☺
Zinc:	9 ☺
MSM:	10 ☺
Apple cider vinegar:	8 ☺

Above are the things I take that work for me, other thing work as well, but these are the best ones for me. Please don't take any until consulting with your doctor or health worker. Some of these made me sick to start, the vinegar was quite hard to stomach, and in my case it took me a while to get use to Garlic, Zinc, and Ginkgo.

It's been a long journey with this disease, one I would not wish on anyone to have to take. Furthermore, I hope by writing my own findings while enduring it, that it may help someone reading my book that has just recently been diagnosed with this disorder. My journey will of course be different, but I hope that some of the things I've found will be of help to you as well. I hope that your doctor or health care provider will work with you, with regards to some of the things that I've discovered.

I found it so very hard initially to walk; I've got other health issues, which made it very hard in my case to start walking any distance. But taking MSM supplement in particular for me, helped to take the edge off the pain a little. I still to this day hurt so very much when walking, I suffer with a bulging lower disc, and Cervical Spondylosis, and have damage in the cerebellum part of my brain.

The cerebellum damage I've had since a car crash over 30 years ago, among other symptoms, makes it hard for me to maintain balance, so coupled with tinnitus, it's quite a job for me to walk. But being the determined so and so that I am, I walk no matter what the cost in pain, and I'm glad I do, because it helps burn of any excess salt.

On the next page, are just a few of the things that I've come across, one way or the other, that are reported to help with Tinnitus, Dizziness, Balance problems, high blood pressure, and many other disorders.

PLEASE NOTE

The information, that you will come across within the pages of my book, are intended for informational purpose only.

Furthermore, under no circumstances is the information in these pages, to be used without your own Doctor, or any other Medical professionals, advice being obtained first. Were all different, and a lot of the information contained in this book could cause serious problems with your health. So please do not use anything mentioned in this book, until you have personally cleared it safe for yourself, with your Doctor, or other professional who cares for you. I cannot be held responsible, if you don't take notice of my written warning.

Coenzyme Q10: Said to be good for blood circulation to the ears, among other Thing's.

Bayberry bark: Reported to alleviate tinnitus symptoms in some people.

Burdock root: Reported to be a blood purifier, and healer, by many users.

Goldenseal: Blood purifier.

Lemons: Reported to be good for a lot of disorders, as well as tinnitus.

Ginkgo Biloba: Reported to be able to reduce dizziness and tinnitus, by increasing blood flow to the ears.

Fresh pineapple: Consumed frequently is said to reduce inflammation.

Garlic: Helps many conditions including tinnitus.

Sea vegetable: Reported to be useful for tinnitus.

Meclizine : Reported to maybe reduce tinnitus.

Hypnosis: Reported as being helpful with your tinnitus.

Meditation: Reported to also be helpful with tinnitus.

Goldenseal is: Thought to be able to relieve tinnitus symptoms.

Ligustrum: Is Reported to be useful for dizziness, tinnitus.

Mullein: Some people have claimed this to relieve tinnitus.

Rosemary: Reported to be useful in treatment of tinnitus.

Avena Sativa: Reported to be useful in treatment of tinnitus,

and also reported to help to reduce high cholesterol levels.

Vertigoheel: Reported to be useful in treatment of tinnitus.

Mistletoe tea: Reported to be useful in treatment of tinnitus.

Plantain: Reported to be useful in treatment of tinnitus.

Grape Seed Extract: Reported to be useful in treatment of tinnitus.

Coptis and Rhubarb: Reported to be useful in treatment of tinnitus.

Eucalyptus Oil: Reported to be useful in treatment of tinnitus.

Mushrooms: Some types are reported to be useful in treatment of tinnitus.

(Calcium
& Vitamin D:)   Reported combined to be useful in treatment of tinnitus.

Major Bupleurum: Reported to be useful in treatment of tinnitus.

Aromatherapy: Reported to be useful in treatment of tinnitus.

Rehmannia Eight: Reported to be useful in treatment of tinnitus.

Sesame: Reported to be useful in treatment of tinnitus.

Black cohosh: Reported to be useful in treatment of tinnitus.

Spinach: Reported to be useful in treatment of tinnitus.

Peanuts: Reported to be useful in treatment of tinnitus.

Maidenhair tree: Reported to be useful in treatment of tinnitus.

Acupuncture: Reported to be useful in treatment of tinnitus.

Sunflower Seeds: Reported to be useful in treatment of tinnitus.

Homeopathy: Reported to be useful in treatment of tinnitus.

Horsetail: Reported to be useful in treatment of tinnitus.

Whole grain: Reported to be useful in treatment of tinnitus.

Lesser Periwinkle: Reported to be useful in treatment of tinnitus.
Massage: Good for stress relief.

Castor Oil: Reported to be useful in treatment of tinnitus.

Passion flower: Reported to be useful in treatment of tinnitus.

L-lysine: Reported to be useful in treatment of tinnitus.

Shrimp: Reported to be useful in treatment of tinnitus.

Fenugreek Seed Tea: Reported to be useful in treatment of tinnitus.

Vitamin E: Reported to be useful in treatment of tinnitus.

Vitamin A: Reported to be useful in treatment of tinnitus.

Vitamin B: Reported to be useful in treatment of tinnitus.

Vitamin C: Reported to be useful in treatment of tinnitus.

Choline: Reported to be useful in treatment of tinnitus.

Zinc: Reported to be useful in treatment of tinnitus.

B12: Reported to be useful in treatment of tinnitus.

Beta-carotene: Reported to be useful in treatment of tinnitus.

Copper: Reported to be useful in treatment of tinnitus.

Magnesium: Reported to be useful in treatment of tinnitus.

Selenium: Reported to be useful in treatment of tinnitus.

Biofeedback: Reported to be useful in treatment of tinnitus.

Crab: Reported to be useful in treatment of tinnitus.

Protein rich diet: Reported to be useful in treatment of tinnitus.

Lemon bioflavonoid: Reported to be useful in treatment of tinnitus.

Green Vegetables: Reported to be useful in treatment of tinnitus.

Raw Vegetables: Reported to be useful in treatment of tinnitus.

Raw Fruits: Reported to be useful in treatment of tinnitus.

Almonds: Reported to be useful in treatment of tinnitus.

(Cranio-Sacral Reported to be useful in treatment of tinnitus.
Therapy)

Soybeans: Reported to be useful in treatment of tinnitus.

Shellfish:　　　Reported to be useful in treatment of tinnitus.

Beta 1 : 3 Glucan:　Reported to be useful in treatment of tinnitus.

Neural Therapy:　Reported to be useful in treatment of tinnitus.

Gouda cheese:　　Reported to be useful in treatment of tinnitus.

Vinpocetine:　　Reported to be useful in treatment of tinnitus.

(Unsulfured black:　Reported to be useful in treatment of tinnitus.
strap molasses)

Cypress rosemary:　Reported to be useful in treatment of tinnitus.

Rose oils:　　　Reported to be useful in treatment of tinnitus.

Legumes:　　　Reported to be useful in treatment of tinnitus.

Cooked Beans:　　Reported to be useful in treatment of tinnitus.

Omega-3 fatty acids: Are reported to be very good for tinnitus suffers, and are to be found in the foods below, among others not on the list.

Brussels sprouts

Salmon

Halibut

Cod

Tuna

Flax seeds

Soybeans

Collard greens

Cabbage

Olive oil

Cloves

Kale

Extra virgin olive oil

Walnuts

Kidney beans

Squash

Furthermore, try eating some Vitamin B12 rich foods from a few of the ones in my list below

Beef

Seafood

Oysters

Poultry

Dairy Products

Eggs

The lists I've compiled above, are far from finished, there will be for sure countless other helpful items to be found, and researched. These are just the ones that in my own personal journey, with the disease, I came across that worked for me. In writing my own story down, I really hope that it may help others, if only by seeing that there are many things out there, which can possibly help, but always proceed with the upmost caution. And consult your Doctor before trying anything; it's for your own safety.

Chapter Five

Getting through each day

I never asked to get this disorder, but I need to be tough in mind and body to get through each and every day. No day for me is ever the same, I get good days, these are defined by having reduced ringing sounds in my ears, or fantastic days, defined by no ringing sounds in my ears. Unfortunately for me, fantastic days are very few, but bad days can be defined by the following, if you were to assume 10 to be the highest volume of sound, then I reach and stay with an eight, five to six times a week.

Furthermore, these very loud levels of noise in both of my ears, can keep up for days or weeks, using supplements and other food sources in this book, I can eventually get the upper hand. But it can sometimes take longer than I would wish, and it impacts on my daily life.

I get very sad when my plan of attack does not work, and I'm left with this horrendous all-consuming noise in my ears, it leaves me tearful sometimes. But I've come to learn from eight years of long term suffering, that this is the way it affects me, and I know now when it's going to be bad. One very weird factor, in starting to make my tinnitus problems escalate, is the following.

I've noticed that when the atmospheric pressure changes from either low pressure or high pressure, sunny day to a wet day, or vice – versa, my eardrums, eyes, and head, feel like there filled up with air. Furthermore, I feel like I'm about to explode with pressure at any moment. The pain is off the scale, its crippling; it's like someone pressing my eardrums from inside using their fingers, and also pushing my eyes out of my head. Furthermore, I feel so very sick to the stomach, my ringing sounds in my ears are now top volume of ten, and the headache is the worst you could have.

I don't know if this is because of my other disorder, known as ACM, Arnold Chiari malformation, acquired from a car crash thirty odd years ago, or just my Meniere's disease or both!. But, I do know that it's the worst thing about my disease, I have to endure. I can hardly function in any normal day to the day things, when the weather decides to change either too high or low pressure. Furthermore, once the pressure system stays one or the other, my pressure in head starts to subside. So, if the atmospheric pressure stays high, or low for a prolonged period, pressure in my head disappears, and I feel great, albeit rubbish still with maybe ringing sounds in ears.

Another complication, that further makes it hard to know if it's my Meniere's disease or not making my ear ringing go super loud, is the fact that I suffer from severe neck and back problems that are called spondylosis, which can cause ringing in the ears. So I have several conditions all of which can cause ringing in the ears. So for me, I have days when all my conditions join together, and give me a nightmarish day or longer, of periods of agony.

I awake most mornings wondering what will greet me with respects to the ringing sounds, I always hope every single day when I awake, that I hear nothing with regards to the noise that is my tinnitus. I also awake hoping not to have the feeling of pressure in my eyes, ears and head, because it always makes for a real bad day, which no pain killer will relieve.

So it's really important that you find out what is causing your tinnitus, because to get correct treatment for this disorder is paramount to getting some kind of relief for yourself. I am very unlucky to have several disorders, and a disease that all give rise to the tinnitus, and other symptoms I suffer with daily, so in my case I try to treat each one.

I thought it would be of help, if I wrote down as many disorders that may be related to ringing sounds in the ears, or other noise, and dizziness, and balance problems that I could find. So, in the next few pages I have listed disorders that can cause these symptoms, but would point out, that you will need to consult your own Doctor, to see what it is that's causing your own medical problems. And don't worry, some of the ones listed are really scary ones, but in the main, most people won't be suffering from them. My list will not cover every single disorder, but is as much information that I could gather up.

Each disorder I have listed, has been listed in brief, you will be able to find out in each case more if you so desire. So here they are in no particular order.

Meniere's disease: This disorder of the inner ear, will affect balance, hearing, cause Vertigo, and can give rise to tinnitus, or other types of unwanted noise in one or sometimes both ears. These are just some of the symptoms; you will be able to find out more.

Tea: Taken in high consumption, Can also cause tinnitus.

Coffee: Taken in high consumption, Can also cause tinnitus.

Alcohol: Taken in high consumption, Can also cause tinnitus.

Soda: Taken in high consumption, Can also cause tinnitus.

Allergies: Can also cause tinnitus among other things.

Strong antibiotics: Can also cause tinnitus among other things, to list a few bleomycin, gentamicin, erythromycin, vancomycin, chloramphenicol.

Syphilis: Can also for some people result in tinnitus.

Herpes: Can also for some people result in tinnitus.

Meningitis: Can also for some people result in tinnitus.

Influenza: Can also cause tinnitus among other things.

Mononucleosis: In some people have been found to cause tinnitus.

Measle: In some people have been found to cause tinnitus.

Mumps: In some people have been found to cause tinnitus.

Sudden loud noise: Can also result in tinnitus, among other things.

Viral labyrinthitis: Can also cause tinnitus among other things.

Anti-inflammatories: High dose can give ringing in the ears.

Diuretics: drugs to increase urination can give you tinnitus.

A cold or virus: Can also cause tinnitus among other things.

Otitis media: Inflammation in the ear, which causes ear infection, can feel fullness of the ear, and pressure, can give rise to tinnitus.

TMJ: Which is the disorder known as Temporomandibular joint disorder, can also give rise to ringing in the ears, among other things.

Aging: Just the natural process of growing older can give rise to Tinnitus, at some kind of level, for some of us.

Ear Trauma: We can damage our own hearing, and get Tinnitus, from listening to very loud music, at a concert, or by being in close proximity to road works, or any other extreme noise, we must all take care not to allow our ears to be damaged by noise.

Hypertension: Or high blood pressure can cause Tinnitus.

Hypothyroidism: And low levels of thyroid hormone production.

Neurofibromatosis: Can cause Tinnitus.
Anemia: Can also cause Tinnitus.

Overactive thyroid: Can cause Tinnitus.

Atherosclerosis: Hardening of the arteries can cause Tinnitus.

Quinine: taken for malaria: Taken for malaria can cause Tinnitus.

Cancer treatments: Can also cause tinnitus among other things.

Asprin: Taken for pain, can cause tinnitus.

Chloroquine: Taken for Malaria can cause Tinnitus.

Earwax blockage: Can also cause tinnitus among other things.

Stress: Can also cause tinnitus among other things.

Depression: Can also cause tinnitus among other things.

Neck injuries: Can also cause tinnitus among other things.

Otosclerosis: A fixation of a tiny stirrup bone in your middle ear, can lead to tinnitus.

My list above is by no means complete, there are many more I would think, just wanted to give a good idea of what can cause this disorder. It certainly changed my life for good; I live with this daily, and wish with every heart beat that it will go away. But I will never give into it or let it ever run my life again, like I did in the early days.

I really hope that there is something however small in my book, that will help some of you out there in the same position as me, and that it may ease your burden. The idea of the lists, are for you to maybe go out on the internet, and through search engines, find more out about some of the disorders I've briefly written about here, or check some books out at of your local library maybe.

Taking control, and taking action, is the best way forward, it's easy to try a few things out, get down because they don't work, (I know that was me in the early days) but don't let it get you down, check out daily if possible for any news about tinnitus relief, or anything that may help your own personal situation. And of course, check everything with your doctor first, be sure its ok for you, we don't want to make ourselves worse.

Above all share your problem with family members, your other half, friends, don't sit alone, because with this disorder you will feel very alone anyway, you're the only one who can hear the sounds, so you need support. A problem shared is indeed a problem halved, so seek support from everywhere you can think of.

I actually went on the internet, and found a sound that was almost identical to the one I hear in both my ears, and then played it to my wife, so as to let her have an idea of our awful it was for me. I feel that it helped her better to know what I was going through, and it made me feel a little bit better, by now knowing, that my wife knew what it sounded like. Of course my wife knew already, by the way I had looked, that I'm having a very bad time, but all the same, it was kind of nice knowing she had actually heard the sound I suffer with as well.

That's the worst thing about this disorder, no one but you can hear the noise going on in your ears, so you really do feel isolated in many ways. I can be outside walking on a beautiful sunny day, in a peaceful place like a park, and my ears will be waging sounds like a World War breaking out. Totally ruins so many days, but that's this disorder for you.

One of my pet hates about this disorder, is what happens to me when I'm in a supermarket or anywhere that as lines of shelving. When walking between the isles of a supermarket, the simple act of walking by the shelving makes my head go into a spin, which in turn can give me vertigo. My head will start to feel fuzzy, and then my stomach will churn, I feel like I'm floating, and then the room I'm in starts to spin.

These days I have stopped this from occurring, by looking at the floor, rather than the shelving. It helped me a lot by doing this, and I now do the same thing when faced with rows of anything.

Another problem, a potentially life threatening one for me, is when walking along on a pavement, at any time with no warning, I can suddenly stumble to either the right or left, and many times now have narrowly missed being run over by a bus or car. It scares the life out of me when walking close to a road, so I proceed with great caution.

My wife looks out for me all of the time when were out walking, especially if near cliffs, not that we go near any, I'm so scared just in case I stumble at the wrong time. What made me laugh so much, while writing this book, was my tinnitus as not stopped even for a single hour, it's like it knows I'm writing about it.

I am going to end this book now, and would like to wish every single one of you, the very best of luck, with your journey with this disorder. And wish you all; very soon to be back in the very best of health that you each can achieve.

Thanks so much for buying this book

Michael John Darracott

Please visit my web site to see what other books I've published,
and for details of other books I'm still working on
that are near completion.

www.mikedarracott.com

Thanks for buying my book.

Make notes here